MW01115445

This Notebook Belongs To

____

Made in the USA
Columbia, SC
28 January 2022

54947669R00074